The Definitive

Slow Cooker Recipe book

Easy and Super Tasty Fish and

Seafood

Donna Conway

implied. readers acknowledge that the author is not engaging in the rendering of legal, financial, medical or professional advice. the content within this book has been derived from various sources. please consult a licensed professional before attempting any techniques outlined in this book.

by reading this document, the reader agrees that under no circumstances is the author responsible for any losses, direct or indirect, which are incurred as a result of the use of information contained within this document, including, but not limited to, — errors, omissions, or inaccuracies.

Table of Contents

Baked Cod

Preparation time: 15 minutes

Cooking time: 5 hours

Servings: 2 people

Ingredients:

- 2 cod fillets

- 2 teaspoons cream cheese

- 2 tablespoons bread crumbs

- 1 teaspoon salt

- ½ teaspoon cayenne pepper

- 2 oz Mozzarella, shredded

Directions:

1. Sprinkle the cod fillets with cayenne pepper and salt. Put the fish in the slow cooker. Then top it with

cream cheese, bread crumbs, and mozzarella. Close the lid and cook the meal for 5 hours on low. Serve.

Nutrition:

Calories: 210

Protein: 29.2g

Carbs: 6.2g

Fat: 7.6g

Cod Sticks

Preparation time: 15 minutes

Cooking time: 1 hour & 30 minutes

Servings: 2 people

Ingredients:

- 2 cod fillets

- 1 teaspoon ground black pepper

- 1 egg, beaten

- 1/3 cup breadcrumbs

- 1 tablespoon coconut oil

- ¼ cup of water

Directions:

1. Cut the cod fillets into medium sticks and sprinkle with ground black pepper. Dip or soak the fish in the beaten egg, then coat in the breadcrumbs.

2. Pour water into the slow cooker. Add coconut oil and fish sticks. Cook the meal on high for 1 hour and 30 minutes. Serve.

Nutrition:

Calories: 254

Protein: 25.3g

Carbs: 13.8g

Fat: 11g

Hot Salmon and Carrots

Preparation time: 15 minutes

Cooking time: 3 hours

Servings: 2 people

Ingredients:

- 1-pound salmon fillets, boneless

- 1 cup baby carrots, peeled

- ½ teaspoon hot paprika

- ½ teaspoon chili powder

- ¼ cup chicken stock

- 2 scallions, chopped

- 1 tablespoon smoked paprika

- A pinch of salt and black pepper

- 2 tablespoons chives, chopped

Directions:

1. In your slow cooker, mix the salmon with the carrots, paprika, and the other ingredients, toss, put the lid on and cook on low for 3 hours. Divide the mix between plates and serve.

Nutrition:

Calories: 193

Fat: 7g

Carbs: 6g

Protein: 6g

Chili-Rubbed Tilapia

Preparation time: 15 minutes

Cooking time: 4 hours

Servings: 4 people

Ingredients:

- 2 tablespoons chili powder

- ½ teaspoon garlic powder

- 1-pound tilapia

- 2 tablespoons lemon juice

- 2 tablespoons olive oil

Directions:

1. Place all ingredients in a mixing bowl. Stir to combine everything. Marinate in the fridge within 15 minutes.

2. Get a foil and place the fish, including the marinade, in the middle of the foil. Fold the foil and crimp the edges to seal. Place inside the slow cooker—cook on high for 2 hours or on low for 4 hours.

Nutrition:

Calories: 183

Carbs: 2.9g

Protein: 23.4g

Fat: 11.3g

Fish Mix

Preparation time: 15 minutes

Cooking time: 2 hours & 30 minutes

Servings: 4 people

Ingredients:

- 4 white fish fillets, skinless and boneless

- ½ teaspoon mustard seeds

- Salt and black pepper to the taste

- 2 green chilies, chopped

- 1 teaspoon ginger, grated

- 1 teaspoon curry powder

- ¼ teaspoon cumin, ground

- 2 tablespoons olive oil

- 1 small red onion, chopped

- 1-inch turmeric root, grated

- ¼ cup cilantro, chopped

- 1 and ½ cups of coconut cream

- 3 garlic cloves, minced

Directions:

1. Heat a slow cooker with half of the oil over medium heat, add mustard seeds, ginger, onion, garlic, turmeric, chilies, curry powder, and cumin, stir and cook for 3-4 minutes.

2. Add the rest of the oil to your slow cooker, add spice mix, fish, coconut milk, salt, pepper, cover, and cook on High for 2 hours and 30 minutes. Divide into bowls and serve with the cilantro sprinkled on top.

Nutrition: Calories: 500 Fat: 34g Carbs: 13g Protein: 44g

Chili Bigeye Jack (Tuna)

Preparation time: **15 minutes**

Cooking time: 3 hours & 30 minutes

Servings: 4 people

Ingredients:

- 9 oz tuna fillet (bigeye jack), roughly chopped

- 1 teaspoon chili powder

- 1 teaspoon curry paste

- ½ cup of coconut milk

- 1 tablespoon sesame oil

Directions:

1. Mix curry paste plus coconut milk and pour the liquid into the slow cooker. Add tuna fillet and sesame oil. Then add chili powder. Cook the meal on high for 3 hours and 30 minutes. Serve.

Nutrition:

Calories: 341

Protein: 14.2g Carbs: 2.4g

Fat: 31.2g

Cod and Broccoli

Preparation time: 15 minutes

Cooking time: 3 hours

Servings: 2 people

Ingredients:

- 1-pound cod fillets, boneless

- 1 cup broccoli florets

- ½ cup veggie stock

- 2 tablespoons tomato paste

- 2 garlic cloves, minced

- 1 red onion, minced

- ½ teaspoon rosemary, dried

- A pinch of salt and black pepper

- 1 tablespoon chives, chopped

Directions:

1. In your slow cooker, mix the cod with the broccoli, stock, tomato paste, and the other ingredients, toss, put the lid on and cook on low for 3 hours. Divide the mix between plates and serve.

Nutrition:

Calories: 200

Fat: 13g

Carbs: 6g

Protein: 11g

Thyme Mussels

Preparation time: 15 minutes

Cooking time: 2 hours & 30 minutes

Servings: 2 people

Ingredients:

- 1-pound mussels

- 1 teaspoon dried thyme

- 1 teaspoon ground black pepper

- ½ teaspoon salt

- 1 cup of water

- ½ cup sour cream

Directions:

1. In the mixing bowl, mix mussels, dried thyme, ground black pepper, and salt. Then pour water into the slow cooker.

2. Add sour cream and cook the liquid on High for 1 hour and 30 minutes. Add mussels and cook them for 1 hour on high or until the mussels are opened. Serve.

Nutrition:

Calories: 161

Protein: 14.5g

Carbs: 5.9g

Fat: 8.6g

Seabass Balls

Preparation time: 15 minutes

Cooking time: 2 hours

Servings: 4 people

Ingredients:

- 1 teaspoon ground coriander

- ½ teaspoon salt

- 2 tablespoons flour

- ½ cup chicken stock

- 1 teaspoon dried dill

- 10 oz seabass fillet

- 1 tablespoon sesame oil

Directions:

1. Dice the seabass fillet into tiny pieces and mix with salt, ground coriander, flour, and dill. Make the medium size balls. Preheat the skillet well. Add sesame oil and heat it until hot.

2. Add the fish balls and roast them on high heat for 1 minute per side. Then transfer the fish balls to the slow cooker. Arrange them in one layer. Add water and close the lid. Cook the meal on high for 2 hours. Serve.

Nutrition:

Calories: 191

Protein: 16.6g

Carbs: 3.2g

Fat: 12.2g

Asian Shrimps

Preparation time: 15 minutes

Cooking time: 3 hours

Servings: 2 people

Ingredients:

- ½ cup chicken stock

- 2 tablespoons soy sauce

- ½ teaspoon sliced ginger

- ½ pound shrimps, cleaned and deveined

- 2 tablespoons rice vinegar

- 2 tablespoons sesame oil

- 2 tablespoons toasted sesame seeds

- 2 tablespoons green onions, chopped

Directions:

1. Place the chicken stock, soy sauce, ginger, shrimps, and rice vinegar in the slow cooker. Give a good stir.

2. Cook on high within 2 hours or on low for hours. Sprinkle with sesame oil, sesame seeds, and chopped green onions before serving.

Nutrition:

Calories: 352

Carbs: 4.7g

Protein: 30.2g

Fat: 24.3g

Mashed Potato Fish Casserole

Preparation time: 15 minutes

Cooking time: 5 hours

Servings: 4 people

Ingredients:

- 1 cup potatoes, cooked, mashed

- 1 egg, beaten

- ½ cup Monterey Jack cheese, shredded

- 1 cup of coconut milk

- 1 tablespoon avocado oil

- ½ teaspoon ground black pepper

- 7 oz cod fillet, chopped

Directions:

1. Brush the slow cooker bottom with avocado oil. Then mix chopped fish with ground black pepper and put in the slow cooker in one layer.

2. Top it with mashed potato and cheese. Add egg and coconut milk. Close the lid and cook the casserole on low for 5 hours. Serve.

Nutrition:

Calories: 283

Protein: 16.9g

Carbs: 9.8g

Fat: 20.7g

Chili Catfish

Preparation time: 15 minutes

Cooking time: 6 hours

Servings: 4 people

Ingredients:

- 1 catfish, boneless and cut into 4 pieces

- 3 red chili peppers, chopped

- ½ cup of sugar

- ¼ cup of water

- 1 tablespoon soy sauce

- 1 shallot, minced

- A small ginger piece, grated

- 1 tablespoon coriander, chopped

Directions:

1. Put catfish pieces in your slow cooker. Heat a pan with the coconut sugar over medium-high heat and stir until it caramelizes.

2. Add soy sauce, shallot, ginger, water, and chili pepper, stir, pour over the fish, add coriander, cover and cook on low for 6 hours.

3. Divide fish between plates and serve with the sauce from the slow cooker drizzled on top.

Nutrition:

Calories: 200

Fat: 4g

Carbs: 8g

Protein: 10g

Onion Cod Fillets

Preparation time: 10 minutes

Cooking time: 3 hours

Servings: 4 people

Ingredients:

- 1 onion, minced

- 4 cod fillets

- 1 teaspoon salt

- 1 teaspoon dried cilantro

- ½ cup of water

- 1 teaspoon butter, melted

Directions:

1. Sprinkle the cod fillets with salt, dried cilantro, and

   butter. Then place them in the slow cooker and top

with minced onion. Add water and close the lid. Cook the fish on high for 3 hours. Serve.

Nutrition:

Calories: 109

Protein: 20.3g

Carbs: 2.6g

Fat: 2g

Tilapia in Cream Sauce

Preparation time: 10 minutes

Cooking time: 5 hours

Servings: 4 people

Ingredients:

- 4 tilapia fillets

- ½ cup heavy cream

- 1 teaspoon garlic powder

- 1 teaspoon ground black pepper

- ½ teaspoon salt

- 1 teaspoon cornflour

Directions:

1. Mix cornflour with cream until smooth. Put the liquid into the slow cooker. Sprinkle the tilapia fillets with garlic powder, ground black pepper, and salt.

2. Place the fish fillets in the slow cooker and close the lid. Cook the fish on low for 5 hours.

Nutrition:

Calories: 151

Protein: 21.6g

Carbs: 1.7g

Fat: 6.6g

Haddock Chowder

Preparation time: 10 minutes

Cooking time: 6 hours

Servings: 4 people

Ingredients:

- 1-pound haddock, chopped

- 2 bacon slices, chopped, cooked

- ½ cup potatoes, chopped

- 1 teaspoon ground coriander

- ½ cup heavy cream

- 4 cups of water

- 1 teaspoon salt

Directions:

1. Put all fixings in the slow cooker and close the lid. Cook the chowder on low for 6 hours. Serve.

Nutrition:

Calories: 203

Protein: 27.1g

Carbs: 2.8g

Fat: 8.6g

Nutmeg Trout

Preparation time: 10 minutes

Cooking time: 3 hours

Servings: 4 people

Ingredients:

- 1 tablespoon ground nutmeg

- 1 tablespoon butter, softened

- 1 teaspoon dried cilantro

- 1 teaspoon dried oregano

- 1 teaspoon fish sauce

- 4 trout fillets

- ½ cup of water

Directions:

1. In the shallow bowl, mix butter with cilantro, dried oregano, and fish sauce. Add ground nutmeg and whisk the mixture.

2. Then grease the fish fillets with a nutmeg mixture and put in the slow cooker. Add the remaining butter mixture and water. Cook the fish on high for 3 hours. Serve.

Nutrition:

Calories: 154

Protein: 16.8g

Carbs: 1.2g

Fat: 8.8g

Clams in Coconut Sauce

Preparation time: 10 minutes

Cooking time: 2 hours

Servings: 2 people

Ingredients:

- 1 cup coconut cream

- 1 teaspoon minced garlic

- 1 teaspoon chili flakes

- 1 teaspoon salt

- 1 teaspoon ground coriander

- 8 oz clams

Directions:

1. Pour coconut cream into the slow cooker. Add minced garlic, chili flakes, salt, and ground coriander.

2. Cook the mixture on high for 1 hour. Then add clams and stir the meal well. Cook it for 1 hour on high more.

Nutrition:

Calories: 333

Protein: 3.5g

Carbs: 19.6g

Fat: 28.9g

Sweet Milkfish Sauté

Preparation time: 10 minutes

Cooking time: 3 hours

Servings: 4 people

Ingredients:

- 2 mangos, pitted, peeled, chopped

- 12 oz milkfish fillet, chopped

- ½ cup tomatoes, chopped

- ½ cup of water

- 1 teaspoon ground cardamom

Directions:

1. Mix mangos with tomatoes and ground cardamom. Transfer the ingredients to the slow cooker. Then add milkfish fillet and water—cook on high for 3 hours. Carefully stir before serving.

Nutrition:

Calories: 268

Protein: 24g

Carbs: 26.4g

Fat: 8.1g

Cinnamon Catfish

Preparation time: 10 minutes

Cooking time: 2 hours & 30 minutes

Servings: 2 people

Ingredients:

- 2 catfish fillets

- 1 teaspoon ground cinnamon

- 1 tablespoon lemon juice

- ½ teaspoon sesame oil

- 1/3 cup water

Directions:

1. Sprinkle the fish fillets with ground cinnamon, lemon juice, and sesame oil. Put the fillets in the slow cooker

in one layer. Add water and close the lid. Cook the meal on high for 2 hours and 30 minutes.

Nutrition:

Calories: 231

Protein: 25g Carbs: 1.1g

Fat: 13.3g

Vegetables and Vegetarian

Cauliflower Mash

Preparation time: 15 minutes

Cooking time: 3 hours

Servings: 4 people

Ingredients:

- 1 head cauliflower, cut into bite-sized pieces

- 5 garlic cloves, smashed

- 4 cup vegetable broth

- 1/3 cup Greek yogurt

- 3 tbsp. butter, cut into cubes

- 2 tbsp. fresh chives, chopped

- 1 tbsp. fresh parsley, chopped

- 1 tbsp. fresh rosemary, chopped

- 1 tsp. garlic powder

- Salt

- ground black pepper, to taste

Directions:

1. In a slow cooker, place the cauliflower, garlic, and broth and stir to combine. Cook, covered for about 2 to 3 hours on high.

2. Uncover the slow cooker and through a strainer, drain the cauliflower and garlic, reserving ½ cup of the broth. Transfer the cauliflower into a bowl, and with a potato masher, mash the cauliflower slightly.

3. Add the yogurt, butter, and desired amount of reserved broth and mash until smooth. Add the herbs, garlic powder, salt, and black pepper and stir to combine. Serve warm.

Nutrition: Calories: 105 Carbs: 5.4g Protein: 5.3g Fat: 7g

Mashed Potatoes

Preparation time: 15 minutes

Cooking time: 2 hours & 30 minutes

Servings: 4 people

Ingredients:

- 6 medium red potatoes, cut into ½-inch thick slices
- ½ cup scallions, chopped
- 1 tbsp. fresh oregano, chopped
- 2 tbsp. extra-virgin olive oil
- 2 tbsp. fresh lemon juice
- 2 oz. feta cheese, crumbled
- ½ cup half-and-half
- ¼ cup fresh parsley, chopped

Directions:

1. In a slow cooker, place the potatoes, scallions, oregano oil, and lemon juice and mix well. Cook, covered for about 2 hours and 30 minutes on high.

2. Uncover the slow cooker. Add the feta cheese and half-and-half and with a spoon until creamy. Serve warm with the garnishing of parsley.

Nutrition:

Calories: 148

Carbs: 21.9g

Protein: 3.8g

Fat: 5.7g

Meat-Free Mushroom Stroganoff

Preparation time: 10 minutes

Cooking time: 5 hours

Servings: 3 people

Ingredients:

- 1¼ lb. fresh mushrooms, halved
- 1 onion, sliced thinly
- 3 garlic cloves, minced
- 2 tsp. smoked paprika
- 1 cup vegetable broth
- 1 tbsp. sour cream
- Salt
- ground black pepper
- 4 tbsp. fresh parsley, chopped

Directions:

1. In a slow cooker, place the mushrooms, onion, garlic, paprika, and broth and stir to combine. Set the slow cooker on high and cook, covered for about 4 hours.

2. Uncover the slow cooker and stir in the sour cream, salt, and black pepper. Serve with the garnishing of parsley.

Nutrition:

Calories: 87

Carbs: 12.2g

Protein: 8.6g

Fat:2.1g

Veggies Ratatouille

Preparation time: 15 minutes

Cooking time: 6 hours

Servings: 4 people

Ingredients:

- 1 cup fresh basil
- 3 garlic cloves, minced
- 1/3 cup olive oil
- 2 tbsp. white wine vinegar
- 2 tbsp. fresh lemon juice
- 2 tbsp. tomato paste
- Salt, to taste
- 2 medium zucchinis, cut into small chunks
- 2 medium summer squash, cut into small chunks
- 1 small eggplant, cut into small chunks
- 1 large white onion, cut into small chunks
- 2 cup cherry tomatoes

Directions:

1. In a food processor, add the basil, garlic, oil, vinegar, lemon juice, tomato paste, salt, and pulse until smooth.

2. Put all the vegetables and top with the pureed mixture evenly in the bottom of a slow cooker. Cook, covered for about 5-6 hours on low. Serve hot.

Nutrition:

Calories: 125

Carbs: 11.5g

Protein: 2.7g

Fat: 8.9g

Colorful Veggie Combo

Preparation time: 15 minutes

Cooking time: 3 hours

Servings: 4 people

Ingredients:

- 1 tbsp. olive oil

- 1 lb. eggplant, peeled and cut into 1-inch cubes

- 1 small zucchini, chopped

- 1 small yellow squash, chopped

- 1 small orange bell pepper, seeded and chopped

- 1 small yellow bell pepper, seeded and chopped

- 1 large red onion, chopped

- 4 plum tomatoes, chopped

- 4 garlic cloves, minced

- 2 tsp. dried basil

- Salt

- ground black pepper, to taste

- 4 oz. feta cheese, crumbled

Directions:

1. In a slow cooker, place all the ingredients except for cheese and stir to combine. Cook, covered for about 3 hours on high. Serve hot with the topping of feta cheese.

Nutrition:

Calories: 203

Carbs: 23.6g

Protein: 8.1g

Fat: 190.3

Friday Dinner Veggie Meal

Preparation time: 15 minutes

Cooking time: 4 hours

Servings: 4 people

Ingredients:

- 2 cans cannellini beans, rinsed and drained
- 1 can tomatoes (diced) with basil, garlic, and oregano
- 1 cup zucchini, chopped
- 1 cup red bell pepper, chopped
- ½ cup Kalamata olives pitted and halved
- 2 garlic cloves, minced
- ¼ cup fresh parsley, chopped
- Freshly ground black pepper, to taste
- 2 tbsp. balsamic vinegar
- 2 tbsp. fresh lemon juice
- 1 cup vegetable broth
- ¼ cup feta cheese, crumbled

Directions:

1. In a slow cooker, place all the ingredients except for cheese and stir to combine. Cook, covered for about 4 hours on low. Serve hot with the topping of feta cheese.

Nutrition:

Calories: 181

Carbs: 27.1g

Protein: 10.4g

Fat: 3g

Spicy Chickpeas

Preparation time: 15 minutes

Cooking time: 6 hours

Servings: 4 people

Ingredients:

- 8 oz. dried chickpeas, soaked overnight and drained
- ½ cup extra-virgin olive oil
- 2 onions, chopped
- 1 (28-oz.) can crushed tomatoes
- 2 carrots, peeled and chopped
- 2 medium potatoes, chopped
- 3 garlic cloves, minced
- ½ bunch fresh cilantro stemmed and chopped
- ½ bunch fresh parsley stemmed and chopped
- ½ tsp. ground turmeric
- ½ tsp. paprika
- ½ tsp. ground cumin

- ¼ tsp. ground coriander

- ¼ tsp. ground cinnamon

- ¼ tsp. curry powder

- ¼ tsp. red pepper flakes, crushed

- Salt

- ground black pepper, to taste

- 1 tbsp. honey

- 3 cups of water

Directions:

1. In a slow cooker, place all the ingredients and stir to combine. Cook, covered for about 6 hours on high. Serve hot.

Nutrition: Calories: 316 Carbs: 40.5g Protein: 9.3g Fat: 14.5g

Meatless Dinner Meal

Preparation time: 15 minutes

Cooking time: 4 hours & 5 minutes

Servings: 4 people

Ingredients:

- 1 tbsp. olive oil

- 1 sweet onion, sliced thinly

- 3 garlic cloves, minced

- 30 oz. canned chickpeas, rinsed and drained

- 1 zucchini, chopped

- 1 cup roasted red peppers, chopped

- 1 cup olives, pitted

- 1 cup vegetable broth

- 1 tbsp. capers

- 1 tsp. dried rosemary

- 1 tsp. dried oregano

- 1 tsp. dried thyme

- 1 bay leaf

- Salt

- ground black pepper

Directions:

1. Heat-up oil over medium-high heat in a skillet and sauté the onions and garlic for about 4-5 minutes. Transfer the onion into the cooker with remaining ingredients and stir to combine.

2. Set the slow cooker on low and cook, covered for about 4 hours. Serve hot.

Nutrition:

Calories: 248

Carbs: 39.6g

Protein: 9.3g

Fat: 6.9g

Greek Beef Stew with Paprika

Preparation time: 15 minutes

Cooking time: 4 to 5 hours

Servings: 4 people

Ingredients:

- 1 tbsp of tallow

- 1 1/4 lb. of beef chunks, boneless cut into small pieces

- 2 green onions finely chopped

- 2 cloves of garlic

- Salt and ground pepper to taste

- 1 tbsp of Italian seasonings

- 1 tsp of sweet ground red pepper

- 2 tbsp of tomato paste

- 2 cups of bone broth

- 1 1/2 cups of water

- 2 Bay leaves

- 2 to 3 tbsp fresh chopped parsley

Directions:

1. Heat-up tallow in a large frying pan on medium-high heat. Sauté the beef, green onion, and garlic with a pinch of salt for 2 to 3 minutes.

2. Add all remaining ingredients and simmer for 2 minutes. Transfer the beef mixture to your slow cooker and stir—cover, and cook on high heat for 4 to 5 hours. Adjust the seasonings and serve hot.

Nutrition:

Calories: 320

Carbs: 25g

Fat: 9g

Protein: 38g

Creamy Lamb Legs

Preparation time: 15 minutes

Cooking time: 5 hours

Servings: 4 people

Ingredients:

- 3 lbs. lamb legs cut into chunks

- 1/2 cup garlic-infused olive oil

- 1 lemon juice

- 1 tsp fresh chopped thyme

- 1/2 tsp fresh chopped parsley

- 1/4 cup water

- 2 cups of Greek yogurt

- 2 eggs from free-range chickens

- Salt and pepper to taste

Directions:

1. Wash the lamb, season with the salt, cover, and leave it in the fridge overnight. Pour the oil into your slow cooker and add the lamb chunks.

2. Sprinkle with thyme and parsley and pour the lemon juice and water—cover and cook on low for 3 hours. In a bowl, whisk eggs, Greek yogurt, and some salt and pepper.

3. Pour the egg mixture over the lamb in the slow cooker. Cover and cook on low within 2 hours. Serve hot.

Nutrition:

Calories: 210

Carbs: 0g

Fat: 13g

Protein: 22g

Grilled Aromatic Beef-Pork Patties

Preparation time: 15 minutes

Cooking time: 8 hours

Servings: 6 patties

Ingredients:

- 2 onions finely chopped

- 1 lb. fresh kale, roughly chopped

- 1 1/2 lbs. ground beef meat

- 1/2 lb. ground pork meat

- 1 large egg

- ½ cup of olive oil

- 3/4 tsp fresh tarragon, finely chopped

- 1/2 tsp cilantro, finely chopped

- salt and ground pepper to taste

Directions:

1. Heat-up oil in a frying pan, and sauté onion and kale with a pinch of salt. Add the ground meat, egg, oil, tarragon, cilantro, salt, and pepper to taste.

2. Sauté for 2 minutes and remove from the heat; let it cool for 10 minutes. Knead the mixture until all ingredients are combined well.

3. Using your hands, shape 6 patties. Grease the bottom of your slow cooker and arrange patties—cover and cook on low for 7 to 8 hours. Serve hot.

Nutrition:

Calories: 219

Carbs: 10g

Fat: 15g

Protein: 12g

Marinated Curry-Spiced Goat

Preparation time: 15 minutes

Cooking time: 8 hours

Servings: 4 people

Ingredients:

- 1 lb. of goat or goat meat

- Juice of 1 lemon (fresh)

- 2 tbsp of curry powder

- 3 cloves of garlic, finely chopped

- 1 fresh ginger root, finely chopped

- 1 medium onion, finely chopped

- 2 tbsp of avocado oil

- 1 tbsp of flour

- 2 red onions, cut into rings

- 1 cup of cauliflower in flowerets

- 1 red chili pepper finely chopped

- 1 tbsp of curry powder

- 1 cup of grated tomatoes

- 1 1/4 cup of goat milk

- Salt and pepper to taste

Directions:

1. Rinse, dry and wrap the goat meat with kitchen paper, and place in a large container. Season generously with salt and pepper.

2. Sprinkle with lemon juice and curry powder, garlic, ginger, and chopped onion. Cover and marinate overnight in the refrigerator.

3. Pour oil into your slow cooker and add goat meat with marinade. Add the onion, cauliflower, red chili, curry powder, tomatoes, and goat milk. Adjust salt and pepper.

4. Close lid and cook on high within 5 hours, or on low 6 - 8 hours. Serve hot.

Nutrition: Calories: 230 Carbs: 25g Fat: 8g Protein: 13g

Mustard Olives with Pork Loin

Preparation time: 15 minutes

Cooking time: 8 hours

Servings: 4 people

Ingredients:

- 1 tbsp of lard

- 1 1/2 lbs. of pork loin cut into small pieces

- 2 medium yellow onions, finely chopped

- 1 cup of olives, pitted and sliced

- 1 large red bell pepper finely chopped

- ½ cup of beef broth

- 1 cup of white wine

- 3 tbsp of olive oil

- 3 tbsp of mustard

- salt and ground black pepper to taste

Directions:

1. Coat your slow cooker with lard. Season pork loin with salt and pepper and add it into the slow cooker. Add the onions, bell pepper, and sliced olives.

2. In a bowl, combine the olive oil, mustard, and white wine and pour over meat and vegetables. Cover and cook on high within 4 hours or on low heat for 8 hours. Serve hot.

Nutrition:

Calories: 135

Carbs: 2g

Fat: 4g

Protein: 22g

Pork Fillets with Mustard - Mushrooms Sauce

Preparation time: 15 minutes

Cooking time: 5 hours

Servings: 4 people

Ingredients:

- 1/2 cup of olive oil
- 6 pork fillets
- 1 dry onion finely chopped
- 2 cloves garlic chopped
- 1/2 lb. fresh whole mushrooms small
- 1 glass of dry white wine
- Sea salt and black pepper
- 2 cups warm water
- fresh oregano finely chopped
- fresh basil finely chopped
- 2 tsp of mustard

- 2 tbsp of flour

- 1/2 cup of beef broth

Directions:

1. Heat the oil in a deep-frying pan with a lid. Sauté the pork fillets with a pinch of salt for 5-6 minutes from both sides.

2. Add the onion, garlic, and mushrooms and sauté for 5 minutes; stir—transfer port fillets in your slow cooker.

3. Pour the wine, add salt, pepper, warm water, oregano, and basil, the mustard dissolved in 1/2 beef broth, and toss to combine well. Cover and cook on low within 4 to 5 hours. Serve hot.

Nutrition: Calories: 393 Carbs: 23g Fat: 17g Protein: 42g

Pork Tenderloin with Creamy Mushrooms Sauce

Preparation time: 15 minutes

Cooking time: 4 hours

Servings: 4 people

Ingredients:

- 1 lb. pork tenderloin

- 1 tbsp of flour

- 1 tsp rosemary, dried

- Sea salt

- ground black pepper

- ¼ cup of olive oil

- 1/2 lb. of white mushrooms, sliced

- 2 cloves garlic, finely chopped

- 1 1/4 cup vegetable broth

- Fresh mint leaves for servings

Directions:

1. Cut the pork into slices. Put the flour and rosemary, add salt and pepper, and pork in a large plastic food bag.

2. Close the bag shake it until the meat is covered well. Pour the oil into your slow cooker and add the pork. Add the mushrooms, chopped garlic, and vegetable broth; stir well.

3. Cover and cook on high within 4 hours. Sprinkle with fresh mint leaves and serve.

Nutrition:

Calories: 450

Carbs: 31g

Fat: 16g

Protein: 35g

Sirloin Steak with Broccoli

Preparation time: 15 minutes

Cooking time: 4 hours & 30 minutes

Servings: 4 people

Ingredients:

- 1 1/2 lb. sirloin steak, thinly sliced

- 1 1/2 cups of beef broth

- 2 tbsp of sesame oil

- 1 tbsp of chili sauce

- 2 of green onions, thinly sliced

- 2 cloves of garlic, minced

- 2 cup of broccoli flowerets

- 2 tbsp of flour

- Sesame seeds, for garnish

Directions:

1. Season the beef steak with salt and ground black pepper. Place the steak on the bottom of your slow cooker and pour the broth, sesame oil, chili sauce, garlic, and sliced green onions.

2. Cover and cook on low heat for 4 hours. Open the lid and spoon 1/2 cup of broth and stir the flour. Place the broccoli flowerets over the beef, and cover with the flour mixture.

3. Cover and cook on high within 20 to 30 minutes. Serve hot with sesame seeds.

Nutrition:

Calories: 250

Carbs: 12g

Fat: 7g

Protein: 37g

Succulent Lamb

Preparation time: 10 minutes

Cooking time: 8 hours

Servings: 2 people

Ingredients:

- 2/3 lb. leg of lamb

- 2 tbsp wholegrain mustard

- 1/3 tbsp maple syrup

- 1 sprig thyme

- 1/4 tsp dried rosemary

Directions:

1. Cut 3 slits across the top of the lamb. Put some garlic
    and rosemary in each slit. Add lamb to slow cooker
    and rub with olive oil, mustard, maple syrup, salt,
    and pepper. Cook for 7 hours on low, add a sprig of
    thyme, then cook for an additional 1 hour.

Nutrition:

Calories: 414

Fat: 35.2g

Carbs: 0.3g

Protein: 26.7g

Lamb with Mint and Green Beans

Preparation time: 10 minutes

Cooking time: 6 hours

Servings: 2 people

Ingredients:

- 1/2 lamb leg (bone-in)

- 1 tbsp ghee, tallow, or lard

- 1/8 cup freshly chopped mint leaves

- 3 cups green beans, trimmed

Directions:

1. Pat the lamb, dry with paper towels, and season it with salt and pepper. Grease the slow cooker with ghee, tallow, or lard, then put the lamb inside.

2. Sprinkle with garlic and mint all over. If it makes you more comfortable, add up to half a cup of water. Cover and cook within 4 hours on high.

3. Transfer the lamb to a plate, then place the green beans on the bottom of the slow cooker. Add the lamb again inside—cover and cook for another 2 hours on high.

Nutrition:

Calories: 525

Fat: 36.4g

Carbs: 7.6g

Protein: 37.3g

Braised Lamb Stew

Preparation time: 15 minutes

Cooking time: 4 hours

Servings: 2 people

Ingredients:

- 1 lb. leg of lamb
- 1/2 cup bone broth
- 1/2 cup white wine
- 1 1/2 carrots, chopped
- 1 tbsp butter

Directions:

1. Rub lamb with salt, pepper, and oil. Brown it in a slow cooker set on high. Set it aside and throw in your veggies in the slow cooker, including onion and garlic to taste.

2. When the veggies have acquired the desired crispness, add in the bone broth and wine. Mix thoroughly. Submerge the lamb legs into the mixture. Cover and cook within 4 hours on high.

Tip: Add rosemary and thyme for extra flavor.

Nutrition:

Calories: 782

Fat: 45g

Carbs: 7g

Protein: 72g

Kerala Lamb Stew

Preparation time: 10 minutes

Cooking time: 6 hours

Servings: 2 people

Ingredients:

- 1 1/3 tbsp coconut oil

- 4 1/2 oz coconut milk

- 1 1/3 bay leaves

- 10 curry leaves

- 4 3/4 oz boneless lamb

Directions:

1. Marinate the mutton with the salt, pepper, chili powder, and other spices desired. In a slow cooker,

heat some coconut oil and fry the mutton, browning it on each side

2. Add bay leaves. Cover and cook on low within 5-6 hours. When simmering starts, add the curry leaves and coconut milk. Cook this for another hour.

Nutrition:

Calories: 284

Fat: 20g

Carbs: 3g

Protein: 22g

Fall-Off-The-Bone Lamb Shanks

Preparation time: 10 minutes

Cooking time: 4-8 hours

Servings: 2 people

Ingredients:

- 1 tsp smoked paprika

- 2 rosemary sprigs

- 2 lb. lamb shanks, seasoned and browned

- 1 tbsp extra virgin olive oil

- 2 organic chicken or beef stock

Directions:

1. Place lamb shanks in the slow cooker. Add the chicken stock; rosemary sprigs, smoked paprika, onions, salt, and pepper to taste into the slow cooker. The meat should be submerged. Cook on high within 4 hours, or low for 8 hours.

Nutrition: Calories: 441 Fat: 27g Carbs: 4g Protein: 19g

Lamb Chops

Preparation time: 10 minutes

Cooking time: 6 hours

Servings: 2 people

Ingredients:

- 4 lamb loin chops

- 1/2 tsp dried oregano

- 1/4 tsp dried thyme

Directions:

1. Prepare the seasonings: oregano and thyme with some garlic powder, salt, and pepper to taste. Rub it on the lamb chops.

2. Put the onion slices in a slow cooker and place chops over the onion slices. Top with garlic, too. Cover and cook within 6 hours on low.

Nutrition: Calories: 201 Fat: 8g Carbs: 3g Protein: 26g

Garlic Lamb Roast

Preparation time: 10 minutes

Cooking time: 10 hours

Servings: 2 people

Ingredients:

- 2 tbsp coconut vinegar

- 1 tsp rosemary

- 1 leg of lamb

- 2 tbsp Worcestershire sauce

- Desired veggies: chopped carrots, onions, and butternut squash

Directions:

1. Put all ingredients in a slow cooker. Add seasonings such as garlic, pepper, and salt to taste. Cook on low within 6-10 hours or until the lamb is tender.

Nutrition: Calories: 435 Fat: 31g Carbs: 6g Protein: 44g

Lamb Shanks with Tomatoes

Preparation time: 15 minutes

Cooking time: 8 hours

Servings: 2 people

Ingredients:

- 1/3 tbsp tomato paste

- 1 x 400g tin diced tomatoes

- 1/3 tbsp sundried tomato pesto

- 1/3 cup beef stock

- 2 lb. lamb shanks

Directions:

1. Heat-up oil in a saucepan and cook onions until translucent. Add garlic and cook for 3 minutes. Add tomato paste and cook for another 2 minutes, stirring.

2. Add diced tomatoes, sundried tomato pesto, and beef stock, then boil. Put the lamb into the slow cooker and pour tomato sauce over—Cook for 8 hours on low.

Nutrition:

Calories: 397

Fat: 34g

Carbs: 5g

Protein: 29g

Lamb Curry

Preparation time: 25 minutes

Cooking time: 8 hours

Servings: 2 people

Ingredients:

- 1 lamb shoulder
- 1 tbsp curry powder
- 1 tbsp ground coriander powder
- 1/2 cup tomato paste
- 1 can coconut cream

Directions:

1. Place lamb shoulder, roughly diced onions, roughly chopped garlic, and 1/4 cup water in the slow cooker. Cover and cook on low for 6 -8 hours.

2. Put the meat aside and add the onions and garlic from the slow cooker to a frying pan. Add curry

powder and coriander powder. Cook until they are integrated.

3. Add tomato paste and cooked lamb meat—Cook for a further 5 minutes. Add coconut cream and simmer within10 minutes on low heat.

Nutrition:

Calories: 554

Fat: 42g

Carbs: 4g

Protein: 28g

Lamb Stroganoff

Preparation time: 5 minutes

Cooking time: 8 hours & 30 minutes

Servings: 2 people

Ingredients:

- 8 oz light sour cream

- 1/8 cup all-purpose flour

- 1/4 cup beef broth

- 1 cup sliced white mushrooms

- 3/4 lb. boneless lamb in 1-inch pieces, browned

Directions:

1. Combine the browned lamb, broth, mushrooms, onions, garlic, salt and pepper, and spices of choice (bay leaf, mustard, or parsley) in a slow cooker. Cover and cook within 6 to 8 hours on low.

2. In a bowl, whisk sour cream and flour until completely integrated. Pour mixture into the slow cooker. Cover and cook on for another 30 minutes on high.

Nutrition:

Calories: 373

Fat: 10g

Carbs: 5g

Protein: 31g

Ground Lamb Casserole

Preparation time: 5 minutes

Cooking time: 8 hours

Servings: 2 people

Ingredients:

- 2 slices bacon, diced cooked crispy

- 1/2 lb. ground lamb

- 1/8 cup chopped green bell pepper

- 2 cups thinly sliced cabbage

- 1 cup tomato sauce

Directions:

1. Add the ground lamb, bacon, pepper, onion, and garlic to taste into the slow cooker. Cover and cook within 6 hours on low. Add the cabbage and tomato sauce to the pot, stir, then cook for another 2 hours.

Nutrition: Calories: 295 Fat: 19g Carbs: 6g Protein: 22g

Lamb Hotpot

Preparation time: 10 minutes

Cooking time: 4 hours & 7 minutes

Servings: 2 people

Ingredients:

- 1 cup lamb stock

- 2/3 lb. diced lamb leg

- 1 1/2 large potatoes in 3mm slices

- 1 large carrot in bitesize pieces

Directions:

1. In a slow cooker, add a little oil plus the onion and carrot. Cover and cook on a low for 5 minutes or until soft but not brown.

2. Change to high, then add the lamb. Cook for 2-3 minutes until browned. Add the lamb stock and a little salt and pepper.

94

3. Arrange the potato slices for them to overlap slightly. Cover and cook within 4 hours on high.

Nutrition:

Calories: 310

Fat: 8g

Carbs: 7g

Protein: 36g

Balsamic Beef Pot Roast

Preparation time: 15 minutes

Cooking time: 3-4 hours

Servings: 4 people

Ingredients:

- 1 boneless (3 lb.) chuck roast

- 1 tbsp Kosher salt

- 1 tbsp Black ground pepper

- 1 tbsp Garlic powder

- ¼ cup balsamic vinegar

- ½ cup chopped onion

- 2 cups of water

- ¼ tsp xanthan gum

For the Garnish:

- Fresh parsley

Directions:

1. Flavor the chuck roast with garlic powder, pepper, and salt over the entire surface. Use a large skillet to

sear the roast until browned. Deglaze the bottom of the pot using balsamic vinegar. Cook 1 minute. Add to the slow cooker.

2. Mix in the onion, and add the water. Once it starts to boil, secure the lid, and continue cooking on low for 3 to 4 hours.

3. Take the meat out of the slow cooker, and place it in a large bowl where you will break it up carefully into large chunks.

4. Remove all fat and anything else that may not be healthy such as too much fat. Mix the xanthan gum into the broth, then add it back to the slow cooker. Serve!

Nutrition: Calories: 393 Carbs: 3g Protein: 30 g Fat: 28 g

Beef Bourguignon with Carrot Noodles

Preparation time: 15 minutes

Cooking time: 5 hours

Servings: 4 people

Ingredients:

- 5 slices - thick-cut bacon

- 1 (3 lb.) chuck roast/round roast/your favorite

- 1 large yellow onion

- 3 diced celery stalks

- 1 bay leaf

- 3 large minced garlic cloves

- 4 sprigs of fresh thyme

- 1 lb. sliced white button mushrooms

- 1 tbsp. tomato paste

- 1 cup Beef/chicken broth (+) more as needed

- 1 cup Red wine

- 1 large carrot

For the Garnish:

- Chopped parsley
- Salt & Pepper
- Optional: Dash of red pepper flakes

Directions:

1. Prepare the bacon in a frying pan using the med-high setting on the stovetop. Place on a paper towel to drain the grease.

2. Flavor the beef cubes with pepper and salt to taste. Layer the meat in the skillet, and sear 1 to 3 minutes. Flip it over and sear another 2 to 3 minutes. Toss it in the slow cooker after all of the cubes are cooked.

3. Fold in the bacon, garlic, mushrooms, celery, and onion in the cooker. Push the thyme and bay leaves between the layers. Empty the broth and wine to cover the mixture approximately ¾ of the way up the cooker.

4. Close the top and cook for 4 hours on high. Shred the carrots to make 'noodles' using a peeler. Cover and cook for another hour or until the beef falls from the bone.

5. Trash the bay leaves when the meal is done and mix well. Serve with the parsley and pepper flakes.

Nutrition:

Calories: 548

Carbs: 6g

Fat: 32g

Protein: 50 g

Beef & Broccoli

Preparation time: 15 minutes

Cooking time: 6 hours

Servings: 4 people

Ingredients:

- 2/3 cup liquid aminos
- 2 lbs. flank steak
- 1 cup beef broth
- 1 tsp freshly grated ginger
- 3 tbsp. sweetener - your choice
- 3 minced garlic cloves
- ½ tsp salt
- ½ tsp red pepper flakes - to taste - more or less
- 1 red bell pepper
- 1 head broccoli
- 1 red bell pepper

Directions:

1. Set the slow cooker on low. Slice the steak into one to two-inch chunks. Pour in the beef broth, aminos, and steak - along with the ginger, sweetener, garlic cloves, salt, and red pepper flakes.

2. Cook 5 to 6 hours on the low setting. Slice the red pepper into one-inch pieces, and chop the broccoli into florets. After the steak is cooked, stir well.

3. Toss in the peppers and broccoli on top of everything in the slow cooker. Continue cooking for at least 1 more hour. Add everything together, and sprinkle with sesame seeds for the topping.

Nutrition:

Calories: 430

Carbs: 3 g

Protein: 54 g

Fat: 19 g

Beef Curry

Preparation time: 15 minutes

Cooking time: 5-8 hours

Servings: 4 people

Ingredients:

- 2 ½ lb. chuck roast

- 6 tbsp. coconut milk powder

- 2 cups of water

- 3 tbsp. red curry paste

- 5 cracked cardamom pods

- 2 tbsp dried Thai chilis/fresh red chilis

- 2 tbsp Thai fish sauce

- 1/8 tsp ground cloves

- 1/8 tsp ground nutmeg

- 1 tbsp dried onion flakes

- 1 tbsp ground coriander

- 1 tbsp ground ginger

- 1 tbsp ground cumin

- 1 tbsp granulated sugar

To Serve:

- 2 tbsp coconut milk powder

- 2 tbsp granulated sugar substitute

- 1 tbsp. red curry paste

- ¼ cup chopped fresh cilantro

- ¼ cup chopped cashews

- optional: ¼ tsp xanthan gum

Directions:

1. Arrange the chuck roast in the cooker. Empty the milk, water, fish sauce, curry paste, ginger, cloves, nutmeg, coriander, cumin, your chosen sweetener, the onion flakes, chilis, and cardamom pods.

2. Use the low setting for 8 hours or high for 5 hours. Right before serving, arrange the meat on a plate. Whisk the sauce with two tablespoons of the milk

powder, the xanthan gum, sugar substitute sweetener, and curry paste.

3. Tear the meat to shreds, and stir into the sauce. Garnish with some cilantro, and serve.

Nutrition:

Calories: 351

Protein: 26.0g

Carbs: 5g

Fat: 22g

Beef Dijon

Preparation time: 15 minutes

Cooking time: 4 hours

Servings: 4 people

Ingredients:

- 4 (6 oz.) small round steaks

- 2 tbsp steak seasoning - to taste

- 2 tbsp avocado oil

- 2 tbsp peanut oil

- 2 tbsp balsamic vinegar/dry sherry

- 4 tbsp. large chopped green onions/small chopped onions for the garnish - extra

- 1/4 cup whipping cream

- 1 cup fresh cremini mushrooms - sliced

- 1 tbsp. Dijon mustard

Directions:

1. Warm up the oils using the high heat setting on the stovetop. Flavor each of the steaks with pepper and arrange to a skillet. Cook 2 to 3 minutes per side until done.

2. Place into the slow cooker. Pour in the skillet drippings, half of the mushrooms, and the onions. Cook on the low setting for 4 hours. When the cooking time is done, scoop out the onions, mushrooms, and steaks to a serving platter.

3. In a separate dish, whisk together the mustard, balsamic vinegar, whipping cream, and the steak drippings from the slow cooker.

4. Empty the gravy into a gravy server and pour over the steaks. Enjoy with some brown rice, riced cauliflower, or potatoes.

Nutrition: Calories: 535 Carbs: 5.0 g Fat: 40g Protein: 39 g

Beef Ribs

Preparation time: 15 minutes

Cooking time: 6 hours

Servings: 4 people

Ingredients:

- 3 lb. beef back ribs
- 1 tbsp sesame oil
- 1 tbsp rice vinegar
- 1 tbsp hot sauce
- 1 tbsp honey
- 1 tbsp garlic powder
- 1 tbsp kosher salt
- ½ tsp black pepper
- 1 tbsp. potato starch/ cornstarch
- ¼ cup light soy sauce

Directions:

1. Arrange the ribs in your slow cooker. Whisk the rest of the ingredients together, but omit the cornstarch for now.

2. Pour the mixture over the ribs, making sure the sauce covers all sides. Use the low setting and cook for 6 hours. It will be fall off the bone tender.

3. Prepare the oven to 200°F. Move the ribs to a baking pan, and cover with foil to keep warm. Use a strainer to pour the liquid from the slow cooker into a saucepan.

4. Use the high setting and whisk in the cornstarch with a little bit of cold water.

5. Continue cooking - whisking often - just until the sauce has thickened into a glaze - usually about 5 to 10 minutes. Brush the glaze over the ribs and serve.

Nutrition: Calories: 342 Carbs: 7 g Fat: 27g Protein: 23 g

www.ingramcontent.com/pod-product-compliance
Lightning Source LLC
Chambersburg PA
CBHW071112030426
42336CB00013BA/2045